"Holding Cancer in My Hand"
A Learning Everywhere® Experience

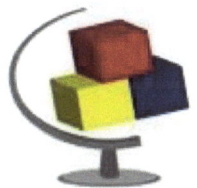

Written by Sheila Stenhouse Lee

"Holding Cancer in My Hand"
A Learning Everywhere® Experience

Written by Sheila Stenhouse Lee

"Holding Cancer in My Hand"
A Learning Everywhere® Experience

In Loving Memory of

Juanita Elizabeth Sykes Stenhouse

My mother, my mentor, my friend.

∞∞∞∞∞∞∞∞∞∞∞∞∞∞∞

"Father, I stretch my hands to Thee,
No other help I know.
If Thou withdraw Thyself from me,
Ah! whither shall I go?"

Charles Wesley

Written by Sheila Stenhouse Lee

"Holding Cancer in My Hand"
A Learning Everywhere® Experience

Create Space is a DBA of On-Demand Publishing LLC, part of the Amazon group of companies. Neither Create Space, Amazon or any of its affiliates endorses this book.

Written by Sheila Stenhouse Lee

"Holding Cancer in My Hand"
A Learning Everywhere® Experience

Contents

Our Story	13
What did you say	14
Never a broken bone	19
Here we go	24
How is it I go	31
Burn that DNR	36
Why are you treating me like this	38
What's going on	42
I talked to god	45
Yard by yard	48
I'm so tired, but I must keep going	51
Coke or Pepsi	59
Self Help	66
Vial of life	67
Pre-paid Funeral Plans	68
(Sample) Last Will and Testament	69
(Sample) Health Care Proxy	72
(Sample) Do Not Resuscitate Order	75
(Sample) Contract for Independent Home Care	77
(Sample) Contract for in Home Physical Therapy	82
Important Contacts	87
List of Medications	88
Prescription Schedule	89
Items to Have on Hand	91
Health Care Journal	92
Accounts Payable	93
Important Papers	95
Glossary	97
Terms A-Z	98

Written by Sheila Stenhouse Lee

"Holding Cancer in My Hand"
A Learning Everywhere® Experience

Acknowledgements

Let me first say thank you to my editors, one of whom Gertrude referred to as my friend with the "educated heart." They ensured this book was written with the clarity, humor and correct grammar and punctuation that Gertrude would have expected.

Gertrude would want me to say "Thank You" to everyone who made this journey as painless as possible, but most of all to say "thank you" for treating her with dignity and respect. I've struggled with whether or not to mention every person by name, but I fear I may forget someone or worse yet spell their name wrong. So let me try this.

There was a women who discovered Gertrude's love for Thai Chi, and shared that passion with her on many an afternoon. Their friendship grew and overtime they had great conversations about many things. She was pleasant yet professional and definitely "sister" material. She in turn introduced me to a team of women who stayed with us through thick and thin.

The Home Health Aides provided Gertrude with the extra love and care when I wasn't able to be there. I never once left her alone or worried a moment about her care or safety. They were her guardian angels here on earth.

Written by Sheila Stenhouse Lee

"Holding Cancer in My Hand"
A Learning Everywhere® Experience

To all of my friends whether you called, clicked or came by. Whether I knew you 3 years or 30, knowing you had my back allowed me to stay strong and to be the woman my mother raised me to be and if you never met her……..not to worry, she lives in me.

To my extended family, many whom I have known since I was a little girl, and my actual family, I feel that it's not my place to say thank you because I know you did it for her more so than for me, but nonetheless I am truly grateful.

So from me to you…………… **I WISH YOU ALL A PEACEFUL JOURNEY**.

Written by Sheila Stenhouse Lee

"Holding Cancer in My Hand"
A Learning Everywhere® Experience

Written by Sheila Stenhouse Lee

"Holding Cancer in My Hand"
A Learning Everywhere® Experience

Foreword

Everyone, regardless of age, race, gender or economic status, has an opportunity to learn something new at any given moment. Sometimes we make a conscientious effort to seek out these opportunities, other times the learning just comes to us out of nowhere. For example, at a conference, in a workshop, or at school, we can anticipate what we are going to learn and the manner in which it will be taught. In those instances we engage in learning so that we can gain new information, skills or strategies that we can apply later. However, every now and then we are blind sided with an experience that is chock full of learning opportunities. Whether welcomed or not, these experiences are thrust upon us most often when we least expect it. The learning that occurs may not be immediately evident, but over time the knowledge gained is recognized.

That is exactly what happened to me. My most memorable and significant learning experience did not happen in a classroom, while attending a conference or while traveling to some remote part of the world. It happened in the home where I grew up with a person who taught me the most, my Mom. This is our learning everywhere experience.

Written by Sheila Stenhouse Lee

"Holding Cancer in My Hand"
A Learning Everywhere® Experience

Prologue

Like many mother and daughter relationships, ours wasn't always the best. We had our good times and bad and sometimes, especially towards the end, the parent-child dynamic was often reversed. That said, our "leaf peaking" trips to Vermont, visits to the cemetery to put flowers on my father's grave, shopping, tea parties or our endless phone conversations about love, life, business and buffoons created a bond like no other.

It was a long time ago when my mother grew weary of me calling her every 5 minutes. "Mom this, Mom that, Mom, Mom, Mom!" I remember being in the bathroom mirror one morning, maybe combing my hair or putting on makeup, with the door open and calling "Mom!" My mother came from the kitchen with fists clenched and a pained expression on her face and she said "if you call my name one more time I am going to scream!" I being a smart-ass said "Ok,' and proceeded to call her by her first name. Juanita. She immediately told me that absolutely was not allowed! "Well-mannered children never called their parents or any other elders by their first name." Yeah, ok I already knew that but, I was feeling kind of "testy." So, I came up with a nickname, "Gertrude," or sometimes "Gerty, Gert." It was a term of endearment that was just ours and ours alone. I've used it ever since. It's funny, when others refer to my Mom as "Gertrude." It's then that I have to correct them and say, her name is "Juanita."

Written by Sheila Stenhouse Lee

"Holding Cancer in My Hand"
A Learning Everywhere® Experience

So this story about Gertrude and I began as a way to help me process things as they were happening, a journal of sorts. However, during Gertrude's final days it was more important for me to be in the moment rather than to capture it. So my notes were put away and I never really thought about them again until much later.

In my travels I have met many people who are now dealing with the issue of aging parents or relatives. Through conversations, Q & As and even some unsolicited advice, I realized that my experiences and the lessons I learned may be a benefit to those who are now walking a similar path. For me, I know a book like this would have been so very helpful with the process, as well as the pain.

That said, I recognize everyone's circumstances, values, beliefs and resources are different. So although this book is in no way intended to be the "end all, be all," it is the story of one mother and one daughter's journey. It will make you laugh and possibly cry, but most of all I hope this in some small way helps you along your journey should there ever be a need.

Written by Sheila Stenhouse Lee

"Holding Cancer in My Hand"
A Learning Everywhere® Experience

Written by Sheila Stenhouse Lee

"Holding Cancer in My Hand"
A Learning Everywhere® Experience

Our Story

A terminal diagnosis is difficult for anyone at any time, but for us it was especially hard as it came out of the blue. Gertrude had indeed slowed down a bit over the years, more so due to transportation issues then determination or will. However, when she could she was still active in water aerobics, Thai Chi and often walked a mile or so several times a week. Her worse vice was her love for Tootsie Rolls® and black jelly beans. I would have sworn she would have out lived all of us, but that was not to be the case.

"Our Story" is not intended as a substitute for the medical advice of physicians. The reader should consult a physician in matters relating to his/her health and particularly with respect to any symptoms that may require medical diagnosis or attention.

"Our Story" is my story, my account of what happened. It in no way is intended to reflect the opinions or experiences of any person other than my mother and me. If anyone should remember similar circumstances, including times, dates, places and people differently than that is their story to tell. Therefore, conversations and locations related herein have been recreated for the sole purpose intended. Any characters mentioned who bear a resemblance to known persons is purely coincidental.

Written by Sheila Stenhouse Lee

"Holding Cancer in My Hand"
A Learning Everywhere® Experience

Chapter I

"What did you say?"

Gertrude was a Tootsie Roll® junkie, a chocoholic of sorts. Seriously, she kept Tootsie Rolls® under her bed pillow in case she needed a fix in the middle of the night. When she was no longer mobile and she would ask that you hand her some, she would get very offended and would tell you so if you only gave her a few. Filling up her whole hand with Tootsie Rolls® until they were falling on the bed for later stashing under the pillow, would always get you a "now that's more like it" and a smile.

On June 26, 2010 after a week of what we thought was severe acid reflux from too much chocolate, Gertrude was diagnosed with stage 4 (terminal) esophageal cancer. This is how we found out.

Gertrude's primary care physician wrote an order for an Endoscopy. A procedure that uses a small, flexible lighted tube to exam the GI tract. On the day the Endoscopy was scheduled we went to the hospital for the simple outpatient procedure. The doctor who performed the Endoscopy and whom we had never met before, turned from one patient's bed in recovery to Gertrude's and without so much as a "Hi, how are you?" said "I performed an Endoscopy on your mother this morning and I found a tumor at the bottom of her esophagus. It's cancer and it's Stage 4." He then said, "Excuse me, my cell phone is ringing. I have to get this," and he walked

Written by Sheila Stenhouse Lee

"Holding Cancer in My Hand"
A Learning Everywhere® Experience

away. At that point I didn't even know how many stages cancer had, but his tone had left me cold. A few minutes later as he finished his call he sat down and started typing away on a nearby computer. "Excuse me" I said, "I know this is routine for you, but as we are hearing this for the first time I need you to go through it in a little more detail as I will have to explain this a million times to family and friends." He repeated it again, with no more compassion than before, but added an operation was not an option because of Gertrude's age (84). We could consider chemotherapy and radiation, but he would let us know what "they" decided after further tests. My Mom nor I are the type of people to have things decided for us, but at that point I was in shock. I couldn't, didn't react. My mother lying in a bed close by looked so hurt and confused. I asked her if she had heard any of what the doctor said and she said "Yes, I think so. I have cancer?" It was at the moment that the reserve that the shock had created for me started to fall away and my blood began to boil. I thought to myself "you will not treat my mother this way!" Little did I know it was only the beginning and things were going to get a whole lot worse.

Over the next few days Gertrude had a Computerized Axial Tomography (CAT) scan and was seen, poked and prodded by a legion of doctors. We would often go to the appointments, me, her and the Home Health Aide in our own car because she disliked ambulances so much. Gertrude said they jostled and bumped her around and she didn't like it

During the first few days after diagnosis she was hospitalized for testing and the doctor who gave the

Written by Sheila Stenhouse Lee

"Holding Cancer in My Hand"
A Learning Everywhere® Experience

initial diagnosis stopped by while 'we' were in the bathroom. "We" being Gertrude, me, the walker, and the IV pole. I couldn't close the door as the bathroom was only slightly larger than a port-o-potty, so the doctor took the liberty of coming to the open doorway and trying to talk to Gertrude while she was on the commode! I immediately cut him off and asked that he come back later. He was very nonchalant as he turned away and said "sure, no problem." He hid out at the nurse's station and only dared return after I had gone downstairs to the cafeteria. Gertrude couldn't recall exactly what he said, but in essence she said "the doctor with the tan hair (he was bald) was here and I don't want him touching me again." Enough said.

Later Gertrude told me she would go as far as she could for as long as she could and in turn I promised I would be with her every step of the way.

Gertrude was hospitalized again for more tests and for 6 days I kept a vigil at her bedside from 6:30 a.m. (ish) to 9:00 p.m. I learned to get to the hospital early as doctors tend to do rounds pre-dawn when the patient, who is often so medicated or sleepy, are alone and not even sure who they are talking to. I typically would only leave her alone if another family member or friend was present. I assisted the nurses with everything, except drawing blood and changing IVs, but became very adept at silencing the alarm on the IV pump when it would go off randomly because the batteries were low. I did so much that one day one of the Licensed Practical Nurses (LPN) mistook me for a Registered Nurse (RN).

Written by Sheila Stenhouse Lee

"Holding Cancer in My Hand"
A Learning Everywhere® Experience

I learned how important it was to stay on top of things by asking "What are you doing," "Why are you doing it," and "Who authorized it?" Once, during that stay, a male nurse came in to take blood which he said he would have to do from the back of Gertrude's hand because of the nature of the lab work to be conducted. He was unsuccessful and caused a lot of pain as he made several attempts with several needles. Later in the hallway he apologized for what I thought was his ineptness, but indeed he was apologizing because he realized later it was the patient in the other bed from whom he was supposed to draw blood.

Towards the end of this stay Gertrude became more than a little bored with the "Thicken" diet (a thickener added to juices to increase the nutritional value) and began to ask for some meat and potatoes. Actually, it was more like a cadence. I asked the nurses when we might be able to start planning to be discharged so Gertrude could eat. We were advised "When she can start to ingest life-sustaining nutrition." Meaning pure liquids or soft food. With unmistaken sarcasm, I in turn suggested if they gave us some "life-sustaining nutrition" than perhaps we could get started! That evening they brought her a mountain of mashed potatoes and some left over ground beef which I recognized from the taco lunch they had served in the cafeteria earlier that day. Gertrude and I, the patient in the adjoining bed and half of the nursing staff could have eaten dinner from that one plate. Gertrude ate a few bites and quickly got discouraged, but

Written by Sheila Stenhouse Lee

"Holding Cancer in My Hand"
A Learning Everywhere® Experience

it was enough to get noticed. So I began the campaign to get her out of there and it worked. We brought her home the next day which I am sure was a direct result of them being sick of us.

Chapter II

"Never a Broken Bone"

Since Gertrude first fell in the spring of 2008, as a result of her Parkinsonia, she had daily in-home care. However, it was only during the week. She fell a second time in the fall of that same year on a Friday night long after her Aide had left for the day. It's ironic that on the same night I awoke after only an hour and couldn't get back to sleep. I laid awake all night tossing and turning and out of boredom started calling Gertrude at about 7:00 a.m., but she didn't answer. After about two hours and numerous unanswered phone messages, I called for help. She had fallen and laid on the hard wood floor for almost 12 hours before found. When I got to her home later that day she was so stiff and hunched over from being on the floor all night that I had to lay on the floor with my head between her feet so she could see me. Gertrude was taken that time to the hospital by ambulance. Later when she was moved from the Emergency Room (ER) Gertrude told me she had heard my voice over the answering machine, when she was laying on the floor, and it gave her hope that someone would be there soon.

Prior to coming home from that hospitalization, Gertrude was in a Rehabilitation (Rehab) Center for two weeks. After she fell she could not walk on her own and had to learn that motor skill again by doing what the Rehab medical staff described as the "Baptist Bounce."

"Holding Cancer in My Hand"
A Learning Everywhere® Experience

She had missed all of her regularly scheduled doctor's appointments during that time, so towards the end of her two weeks I took her to see her Parkinson doctor to determine if anything needed to change regarding her medications or living conditions. Gertrude and I both really liked this doctor and trusted whatever he would tell us. Because it was not a medical emergency no transportation was provided so we got in my car at the Rehab Center and off we went. But for a few minor adjustments to her meds we were told she was fine and free to go home. Now why did her doctor say that? Gertrude still had to be released from the Rehab Center! Driving back I felt like I was transporting an escapee. With one hand on the wheel and one on Gertrude I was afraid the closer we got to Rehab she might jump out of the car and make a run for it. To ease both of our anxieties I asked if she would like to ride by her house, but she solemnly said "No, if we go there I won't want to go back (to the Rehab Center)."

That same afternoon Gertrude and I were invited to attend the Rehab Center's Medical Review Board meeting where her case would be reviewed. It was down the hall from her room and Gertrude and I were seated at the table before the meeting started. I was surprised to find the Board didn't include her nurse, the Physical or Occupational Therapists who had been working with her. It was a group of medical staff who were simply going through her file. As they went around the table reporting on this and that, they ceremoniously announced at the end

Written by Sheila Stenhouse Lee

"Holding Cancer in My Hand"
A Learning Everywhere® Experience

of the following week they would review her case again. She and I were both heartbroken. I interrupted the proceedings and announced that we had seen her doctor that day. The doctor had made some minor adjustments to her medications and said she could go home. As they probably hadn't received a copy of the doctor's report yet I suggested we give the new prescription schedule a couple of days to take effect. If there were no problems, then we would be taking Gertrude home in a few days. The head "whoever in charge," looked at me and said "Oh, you would like us to review her case at that time to determine if she is ready to go home?" "No," I corrected her. "In the next few days if there are no further issues, she is coming home!" Gertrude was released 3 days later and we got her Life Line (an emergency call button) that she wore around her neck at all times. If there was an emergency she simply had to press the button to be connected over a loud speaker in her home directly to a 911 operator. A hospital bed was also ordered, but when it was delivered it was set up in the dining room. Gertrude insisted quietly, yet quickly, that I have it moved to a bedroom and "get her house back in order!"

  Sometime that spring, Gertrude fell again in the middle of the night. At this point her physical capabilities were greatly diminished. She would sometimes loose her balance and not have the strength to pull herself up off the floor. This was particularly worrisome at night when she needed to use the bathroom. In hindsight adult diapers or a portable commode would

"Holding Cancer in My Hand"
A Learning Everywhere® Experience

have been smart. This time she used the Life Line. I was surprised. Then I realized she was terribly frightened of being on the floor again, all night, cold and alone. When the fire department called me at 3:00 a.m., the firemen who came through the dining room window assured me she was alright and that they hadn't damaged anything. Gertrude refused to go to the hospital. So I called our closest family friend to stay with her through the night.

When Gertrude fell a third time in the summer of 2009 we knew it was time. We increased her Home Health Aides to 24 hours a day, 7 days a week and canceled the Life Line. Her Medical Insurance didn't cover any of it, but some wise investments and aggressive saving made it possible for us to pay almost $10,000 a month out-of-pocket while maintaining all of her other household expenses and medical needs. It was costly, but we did it.

You see, in the state where she lived, a person cannot own any real assets for a period of five to eight years prior to a request for assistance from Medicare and Medicaid. So the message is PLAN AHEAD! Even if Gertrude had liquidated all her assets at the time of her diagnosis, she still would have had to wait another five to eight years before she received any help from the state. This worried her and she would often ask "How much money do I have left?" Fortunately or not, Gertrude still owned and lived in the house she and my Dad had purchased 55 years ago and she was not budging. In fact,

"Holding Cancer in My Hand"
A Learning Everywhere® Experience

she had made me promise many years earlier that no matter what happened we would never let anybody take her from her home.

Written by Sheila Stenhouse Lee

Chapter III

"Here We Go"

On July 9, 2010, after the cancer diagnosis, I received a call from Gertrude's Home Health Aide at about 12 midnight. "I would like to take your Mom to the hospital" she said. When I asked why, she said because Gertrude was saying "she wanted to go home." The Home Health Aide was afraid Gertrude might be a bit delirious from dehydration. I told her that I would call our closest family friend, as I was 5 hours away at my home in Maryland, to come be with Gertrude for transport to the hospital if that is what the Home Health Aide thought was best. Earlier that day, Gertrude had just told me that she did not want to go back to the hospital, but as the Home Health Aides saw her on a daily basis, and could quickly determine a change in her condition, I would follow their lead. About an hour later the Home Health Aide called again and said the paramedics had arrived, but Gertrude refused to go to the hospital. State law dictates that if a person is fully conscious and lucid then paramedics cannot take a person to the hospital against their will. The Home Health Aide said Gertrude's vitals (temperature, blood pressure and oxygen levels) for the most part were good, but her pressure was 190 over 109. I asked to speak with her. I said "Gertrude, I know you don't want to go to the hospital, but your pressure is a little high!" She said "Oh please, your pressure would be high too if you woke up in

"Holding Cancer in My Hand"
A Learning Everywhere® Experience

the middle of the night and there were a bunch of men in white coats standing over your bed!" All I could do was laugh and after she reminded me that sometimes her medicine made her a little "loopy" and that everyone suffers from a little "white coat" syndrome she assured me she was truly alright. What could I do? So we said "good night."

In hindsight, I wasn't surprised that Gertrude regaled the paramedics with her knowledge and wit. At 84 she began every day with a statement of the day and date, her name, address, birth date and social security number. This was followed by a crossword puzzle and rounds of Sudoku throughout the day. Back in November 2008, when Gertrude was in the Rehab Center she made it a point for me to get her an absentee ballot on the day before the national presidential election (as Gertrude wouldn't be home in time to vote). This was a very important election and Gertrude remembered all too well when voting for African Americans was a life-threatening task. So I called a friend who was well versed in the local political process. She instructed me to go to the Department of Motor Vehicles and get an absentee ballot. So off in the snow I went and when I returned to the Rehab Center I had Gertrude's ballot in hand. After putting an "X" next to Barack Obama's name on the ballot Gertrude told me she didn't care about the other folk and I should fill out the rest of the ballot anyway I wanted. Gertrude also made it clear that I was to return to my own voting district in Maryland that night so that I

"Holding Cancer in My Hand"
A Learning Everywhere® Experience

would be home in time to vote the next day. It was late that evening when I returned home, but the next day I was up at 7:00 a.m. to cast my vote. I moved into my first office that day too, so for me on so many levels it was a historic day. By the time Obama's presidency was declared that evening I was exhausted and already in bed sleeping. I missed all the media coverage that night, including the acceptance speech in Grant Park. It didn't matter as somehow I knew from the time Gertrude had voted, Barack Obama had won the election! All that said, when it came to "naming the President" I was sure it was something she would never forget.

Back to 2010. I remember on July 12th I flew back to New York to take Gertrude to a series of doctor's appointments. I had been doing this with Gertrude regularly for the last three years. She always wanted to have someone with her when she went to the doctor's because she wasn't always clear about what they said or what questions she should ask. This required the on-going coordination of my schedule with her Doctor's office staff so needless to say, they knew me well. That day we started with her gerontologist. This doctor who Gertrude referred to not so fondly as "Shorty" was a part of the same practice as the doctor with the "tan hair." When the Doctor came into the examination room with his lap top open, sat it on the counter and began a rapid succession of questions, I did my best to respond just as quickly. He never said "hello," "nice to see you," or even asked "how are you feeling?" At some point Gertrude

"Holding Cancer in My Hand"
A Learning Everywhere® Experience

got very aggravated because she was being talked about, talked around, but not talked to, and she told "Shorty" so. She said something to the effect "if you would direct your questions to "her" and not about "her", "she" would be happy to answer you." "Shorty's" question and answer period came to an abrupt halt. "Shorty" made a few more entries which I am sure included something about the patient's "bad attitude" and left the room. However, before doing so he casually asked over his shoulder "do you need any (prescription) refills?" This was particularly disturbing as he nor his staff ever weighed Gertrude, took her blood pressure or checked her breathing. More importantly shouldn't a doctor's records indicate whether a patient should be ready for a refill or not?

That said, I was well aware that "Shorty" was not a fan and the feeling was mutual. That became apparent a few months earlier when Gertrude first fell and he insisted that she be moved into an assisted living facility or nursing home because "she shouldn't be living alone." When I told him we had 24 hour Home Health Aides, he was quick to tell me "that's very expensive and you probably can't afford that for long." I suggested he "stick to medicine and we would handle the rest." Later when Gertrude shared that "Shorty" was also the Director of the entire assisted living/nursing home network in the area (talk about pushing your own agenda), I quickly dismissed his concern as being totally self-serving.

"Holding Cancer in My Hand"
A Learning Everywhere® Experience

Later that day we went to the Cancer Care Center. What a totally different experience. We were first met by the Patient and Family Care Nurse and then later the doctor. The Doctor was a patient, kind women who sat eye level with Gertrude and spoke directly to her without ever taking a note or consulting a file. This was the type of treatment any person would want and Gertrude deserved. The doctor's office made all the appointments necessary for Gertrude's consultations with other doctors. As we left they gave us a Cancer 101 book and an expandable folder for filing all our documents from the offices we would be visiting. For the first time, and after being diagnosed 2 weeks earlier, we received a "Cancer of the Esophagus" booklet.

Gertrude's cancer was a text book case. Esophageal cancer is a tumor in the area of the heart. Initial symptoms include pain behind the sternum, often a burning, heartburn-like feeling which may be severe and present almost daily, followed by painful swallowing. Fluids and soft foods are usually tolerated, but hard or bulky substances (such as bread and meat) become impossible to swallow over time. As a result there is substantial weight loss as a result of reduced appetite and poor nutrition. Another sign may be an unusually husky, raspy, or hoarse-sounding cough, and drooling. The tumor surface may be fragile and bleed, causing vomiting of blood. Most people diagnosed with esophageal cancer are diagnosed in the late-stage of the disease, because typically there are no significant symptoms until half of the inside of the esophagus, is obstructed, by which point the tumor is fairly large. Tobacco smoking and alcohol use can increase the risk and together may increase the

Written by Sheila Stenhouse Lee

"Holding Cancer in My Hand"
A Learning Everywhere® Experience

risk by more than 90%. Almost everything noted here is something Gertrude experienced at one point or another over the next six months.

To answer your question, yes Gertrude had been a smoker. She had quit sometime in the 1950s so as to hear her tell it "not burn the house down." Apparently she always left the house in a rush and was never sure that she had properly extinguished her cigarette, so she quit. She also loved her cold beer. I don't think she ever would have anticipated that these occasional pleasures would have caused her such harm, but with this information Gertrude and I felt better armed for what lay ahead.

Then all hell broke loose. The night of July 15, 2010, I received a call from the Home Health Aide. Gertrude had started to bleed profusely from the nose and mouth. I told them to call 911 immediately and I called our closest family friend again and asked her to meet the ambulance at the hospital. It was too late for me to get on the road and I was scheduled on a 7:30 a.m. flight the next day anyway to take Gertrude to another medical appointment. I would meet them at the hospital by 9:00 a.m. When I arrived at the hospital the next morning Gertrude was in a room and in good spirits even though she was very perturbed to be out of the house without her glasses and teeth. The bleeding had stopped. She had some old clots which were dark brown in color, which she was spitting up, but for the most part she was doing

Written by Sheila Stenhouse Lee

well. So as her closest family friend left and my friend arrived we were feeling cautiously optimistic.

Chapter IV

"How is it I go to the doctor every 3 months and he didn't know what the (bleep) was wrong with me?"

As I waited at the Nurses station, per their request, to sign consent forms for another Endoscopy (I was Gertrude's Health Care Proxy), my friend came into the hall, arms flailing, telling me to come quick. Gertrude had begun to spit up fresh blood again and it was everywhere. The nurses did not initially follow, but when they did come into the room they told us to "calm down" and "back up" as they made arrangements to do a portable (in her room), chest x-ray, stat (now!) and we were told to leave.

    Gertrude was conscious and anxious to know "what the hell" was going on. Amidst all the confusion and Gertrude's impression of Mount Vesuvius, I was asked to authorize another Endoscopy and Gertrude quickly told everybody she would sign it. My friend and I went to the visitor's lounge to wait and the next thing I knew I was being paged over the hospital intercom. Gertrude had been moved to the Intensive Care Unit (ICU). When we arrived, they were preparing her for the Endoscopy which in her weakened state would require sedation and a respirator. Even though the bleeding had

"Holding Cancer in My Hand"
A Learning Everywhere® Experience

slowed down a bit, Gertrude herself told them to "hurry up!"

For six days we watched and waited while Gertrude was periodically weaned on and off the respirator only to be put under again using Diprivan (Propofol). Sound familiar? As she was not put on the breathing tube for respiratory problems the prognosis was good, but we were asked to prepare for the possibility that she would not breathe on her own again or regain consciousness.

During this time we were told that the blood thinner she had been taking since her previous hospital visit had caused the bleeding and they were taking her off it immediately. The esophagus had been cauterized where the blood thinner had caused damage, but as the occurrence of blood clots were originating in the lungs and not the legs where they could have inserted a filter to stop clots from traveling to major organs, they were going to insert a "basket" to catch the blood clots around her lungs. Now none of this was described with the simplicity that it is here, so when the doctors would explain things in medical terms I would do my best to repeat it in layman's terms to make sure I got it right. Some of the doctors were patient with me, some were not. Numerous doctors came and went. Full color glossy photos of Gertrude's internal organs were shared, but I would often turn away. Questions to medical professionals like "what would happen when the basket

Written by Sheila Stenhouse Lee

"Holding Cancer in My Hand"
A Learning Everywhere® Experience

got full" often went unanswered. So if it hadn't been for another family friend, a retired RN nicknamed by her own family as Nurse Jane Fuzzy Wuzzy, who helped translate much of what was said I surely would have jumped out a window and likely taken someone with me.

The hardest thing during this time was not being able to talk to Gertrude. I could see her and touch her, hold her hand, but I couldn't explain what was happening or get her advice, much less find something silly to laugh about. Sometimes as she was being weaned off the respirator to check her breathing levels and she became semi-conscious, her strangled attempts to speak were excruciating to watch. Visits by family and close friends that were shocked to see her in such a drug-induced state were tough, and the comments from staff about the beauty of her skin, what products she used or how they couldn't believe she was 84 seemed insensitive. She was dying, but she looked good? Seriously!

Gertrude began to bleed again and although the doctor with the "tan hair" was consulted by the ICU staff only by phone, he felt her blood levels were "good enough" to take her off the respirator. The lung specialist however felt that we should wait for another test to be done. In the event the tube was pulled out and had to put it back in it would be very difficult, if not impossible. During all this I had to go back to Maryland for my own medical appointment. In 2008, I had been diagnosed with Multiple Sclerosis and was assigned to a medical

Written by Sheila Stenhouse Lee

"Holding Cancer in My Hand"
A Learning Everywhere® Experience

study group. It was an appointment that could not be missed. It was debated whether further tests should be done and whether or not Gertrude should remain on the respirator until I returned the next day. It was agreed I would go and come back before anything further was done.

As my plane landed in Maryland that night, I received a call from the hospital advising that the doctor with the "tan hair" had finally come to see Gertrude (thank God she was asleep) and decided another Endoscopy should be done. I gave verbal consent for it to happen the next day. However, when I got to my house I called "Nurse Jane Fuzzy Wuzzy" to get her opinion. Even though she thought that it was the right course of action, she reminded me that Gertrude had said she didn't want that doctor to touch her again. She advised I call back to ICU, have the doctor with the "tan hair" taken off the case and get a new doctor assigned. I did that right away and although they called me at 9:00 p.m., still not having identified a replacement, they assured me they would find someone to do the procedure the next day and I should rest well.

The next afternoon, after my own appointment I drove back from Maryland to New York in record time. When I arrived back at ICU I was informed that one of the two specialists who needed to be present for the removal of the respirator (so the Endoscopy could be done again) was already gone for the day. Fortunately,

"Holding Cancer in My Hand"
A Learning Everywhere® Experience

the next morning it was with great relief that the doctor who was to perform the procedure came by to tell us after further test they found no further complications and he was removing the respirator. Another Endoscopy would not be necessary. In total Gertrude had been sedated for a full seven days.

Written by Sheila Stenhouse Lee

"Holding Cancer in My Hand"
A Learning Everywhere® Experience

Chapter V

"Burn that "Do Not Resuscitate" order, Life is worth living!"

On July 21, 2010 the respirator was finally removed and Gertrude was able to breathe on her own. Afterwards a Nurse Practitioner jiggled the bed using an electronic stimulator that rocked and rolled the bed for about a ½ hour to loosen the phlegm from Gertrude's chest. She absolutely hated this procedure and asked repeatedly that it stop. When it finally did she told us, once she found out the day and the date, that it was her and my dad's 60th wedding anniversary. Her mind was as sharp as ever. Even though her throat was sore and her voice very raspy she had a lot to say. In an unfamiliar and gravely tone she summoned everyone in the room close to her bed and asked "how has my (primary care) doctor ("Shorty") seen me every 3 months for years and he had no idea what the "(bleep)" was wrong with me?" As we all laughed, she proclaimed, having established years earlier a Health Care Proxy, Living Willing, Power of Attorney and a Do Not Resuscitate (DNR) order that she wanted to live! "Tear up that DNR, life is worth living!" she said. Gertrude was back. As she got stronger family and friends rejoiced, cried, called and in general celebrated!

Gertrude asked me to stay with her that night in ICU and although I knew it wasn't going to be super comfy, and the one thing I really needed was sleep, I was happy to oblige. The medical staff was very attentive and tended to her every need. This meant they checked on her no less than every two hours. Although care and treatment in ICU far exceeded anything we had ever experienced on a regular floor, it was while there that Gertrude got a bed sore in the middle of her lower back that in her final days required regular dressing and packing. It caused her more pain than the cancer ever would.

    That's when the guilt set in. I felt Gertrude's bed sore was my fault. If I had just canceled my medical appointment in Maryland, Gertrude would have been weaned off the respirator two days earlier. The reality is the cancer was not going to just go away and her body had already begun to break down.

Chapter VI

"Why Are You Treating Me Like This?"

Once back on a regular floor, while other family members sat with Gertrude during the day I went to her house to shower, sleep and get the house ready for her return. I added grab bars everywhere, removed rugs and got new furniture that was more accommodating to her needs. When I arrived back at the hospital at about 4:00 p.m. each day, Gertrude would ask me to stay with her through the night. Even though I was exhausted and wanted to sleep in a bed, I was so often glad I did. I remember years ago while traveling abroad I visited an African hospital. I was surprised to find the hospital waiting area was not filled with "visitors" which is typical in American hospitals, but "guardians." In this African culture a "guardian" comes to the hospital with the patient to attend to their personal needs after the medical treatment is over. In hindsight it's a wonderful idea, based on what I've seen, and one I would highly recommend that every family consider.

On our last night in the hospital, Gertrude went without food or water from 4:00 p.m. until 9:00 a.m. the next morning. If I hadn't given her periodic swipes of a moistened mouth swab she would not had anything at all. During this time she received through an IV drip only an antibiotic, a fluid to flush the catheter and potassium. The only medication she received during the night by

"Holding Cancer in My Hand"
A Learning Everywhere® Experience

medical staff was her eye drops. About 3:00 a.m. I asked for assistance in turning her as she had been in the same prone position, lying on a bed sore for about 12 hours. However, it wasn't until about dawn that my temper really flared.

All night I been by Gertrude's bedside in a chair holding her hand. When she needed something she need only to squeeze my hand to let me know. When she did this at about 6:30 a.m. and told me "Shorty" had been there I thought she had been dreaming. But as I closed my eyes again, she repeated her words. At about 8:30 a.m., I asked the nurse at what time the doctor would do his rounds. She told me he had already been there and left. Even in her weakened state I got the proverbial "I told you so" from Gertrude. I asked, or maybe I told the nurse "to get him on the phone!" She gave me his office number and I called him immediately. He came on the line .... and said: "Yes, I saw your mother this morning." I asked if he hadn't also noticed me in the chair directly next to her bed, holding her hand, and he said "yes, but your eyes were closed." What went through my mind at that moment, and even now, is even the slimiest of snakes makes a noise. I can't clearly remember what he said after that, not because I was overwhelmed, but simply because I stopped listening. His credibility as a medical professional and as a human being was gone. I told him that "they" were not at this point providing anything that we could not offer Gertrude at home. She had 24 hour home health care, a hospital

"Holding Cancer in My Hand"
A Learning Everywhere® Experience

bed, a pill crusher (mortar and pestle), a salvia sucker and a physical therapist. We were taking her home. He told me he agreed with me on a philosophical level, but as Gertrude had recently pulled the DNR order we were suggesting "comfort care," but should the need arise "do all you can." Like his opinion mattered. I told him "to get the discharge papers ready!" He said he would contact her cancer doctor. In closing, I might have said "thank you," but I don't remember, and I don't care.

Shortly thereafter, Mom squeezed my hand again and told me she was hungry. I told her "the breakfast tray should be here soon."

When it didn't come she asked me to take her to breakfast and I told her I couldn't because we would get in trouble. Gertrude, who was always one of the strongest women I know, broke into tears and asked "why are you treating me this way?" It broke my heart. We were both sleep deprived, hungry, desperate and vulnerable and those types of emotions tend to bring out the worst in anyone and it did in me. I went and demanded something to eat for her from the nurses and they knew I wasn't just joking. I was only given two Jell-O size cups of cherry "thicken", but I tried to make the best of it, knowing that this "breakfast" was not going to go over well at all. I felt like I was on a cell block, but I did my best to make it seem appetizing for Gertrude's sake. She was so disappointed and refused to eat it, especially when the patient next to us was given hot and buttery French toast albeit hospital style. Gertrude looked so envious even though she and I both knew she didn't even like French toast.

Thank God at that point the cancer doctor came in and talked to us. Calmed me down was more like it. I explained we were ready to go home because what we had available for Gertrude there was the same or more than we were being offered in the hospital. We were not giving up, just taking a break and the cancer doctor agreed it was the best thing for her. When the Lung Specialist came in and I told her the same, the Lung Specialist also agreed. With their urging, the nursing staff quickly got discharge papers ready, the dietician prepared a grocery bag full of Ensure, "thicken" and dairy supplements, the discharge planner arranged for ambulatory transportation from the hospital to our home and by 3:45 p.m. that same day (Ok, so everything requires a little patience, thanks Gertrude) Gertrude was home.

That night, while the Home Health Aides tended to Gertrude, a friend came and cooked dinner for the family. With the exception of the smoke detector going off a couple of times, it was a quiet first night.

"Holding Cancer in My Hand"
A Learning Everywhere® Experience

Chapter VII

"What's Going On?"

We were all happy to have Gertrude home. The first morning the Home Health Aides had overlapping shifts to make sure everyone knew what to do. Just as they were changing shifts and tending to Gertrude, I heard a noise. As the Aide who was coming on duty crossed the dining room to the bathroom, I yelled out from upstairs, "is everything alright?" She said "yes," and I said "call me if you need me." Soon thereafter I heard a gush of water. At first I wondered if Mom had required so much changing that a tub washing of linens was necessary. Then I realized the water pressure I was hearing was even more than the shower would yield.

As I came down the stairs I noticed the bathroom light was on, the door was open and the Aide's arms were outstretched holding a towel to the sink's faucet. It was like an open fire hydrant! She yelled that the handle had broken off. As she leaned away from the spray while trying to hold the towel in place the bathroom began to flood. I pushed her to the side and began to pull all of my mother's WWII provisions from under the sink to turn off the water, BUT BECAUSE THE HOUSE WAS OVER 50 YEARS OLD THERE WAS NO SHUT-OFF VALVE UNDER THE SINK, so I went down into the dirt cellar. There was so much water it was now raining through the bathroom floor boards. I turned every valve I could find,

Written by Sheila Stenhouse Lee

"Holding Cancer in My Hand"
A Learning Everywhere® Experience

but to no avail. I came back to the bathroom and repeated the process a few times before running upstairs to get my robe and glasses and try again. By now the Aide was soaked, but she diligently remained like a child with her finger in the dam. However, in this case it was at the faucet with a towel. I finally conceded and called 911. They answered the call, but as I paced with the phone I realized that the phone cord had become disconnected from the base. Gertrude had lived in the same house for 55 years, the phone number had been the same and there was no turn off valve under the sink................go figure! At that point I was directly in front of Gertrude's bedroom and she stared me down trying to figure out what the hell was going on. The other Aide sat at her bed side making idle conversation and doing her best to act as if nothing was happening.

    After contacting the neighbors, who had been on the block since I was a child and knew the house as well as we did, looked and couldn't find the valve either, the Fire Department finally showed up and turned off the water main. It was too late. By then we were all soaking wet. The Aide who was in the bathroom the whole time was sent home to change her uniform and I dared to restart my day with some sort of normalcy by taking a shower. It was then that I realized, there was no water! Saturday afternoon, it was 90°, we had just brought home a terminally ill cancer patient and we had no water. Great! Expense was of no consequence at this point, so I

"Holding Cancer in My Hand"
A Learning Everywhere® Experience

searched the yellow pages for a plumber who could come fix the faucet right away …………….. cha ching!!!!

Shortly after the plumber arrived, fixed the sink and turned the water back on, the physical therapist came and began a session with Gertrude. It was important to maintain Gertrude's schedule as much as possible. The therapist wanted all of us who would be a part of Gertrude's daily care to observe her physical therapy session. We all really liked her and knew she had Gertrude's best interest at heart so in turn we did our best to give her our undivided attention ………….Gertrude, me, 2 Home Health Aides, three family members, the plumber and a dog. This particular ordeal made it clear to me that you had to be prepared for anything and everything.

Chapter VIII

"I Talked to God"

I don't know that we ever settled into any kind of routine on that first day, but by the time the sun set, sleep came easy. However, at about 11:00 p.m. I heard another commotion. Gertrude had started choking and was struggling with great difficulty to catch her breath. I told the Home Health Aide to call 911. The gurgling and Gertrude's constricted windpipe created such a violent noise, that at one point I covered my ears. The Home Health Aide said, "call 911?" I shouted "yes, call 911!" and at that point Gertrude looked me in the eye and said in a raspy and weary voice "don't call." I was panicked and clearly it was not a good time for a battle of wills. Gertrude was choking to death. It was then that I remembered when she was weaned off the respirator the nursing staff set the bed to "vibrate" and a Patient Care Attendant (PCT) told me that before modern technology they rolled patients on their sides and patted their backs until they coughed up the phlegm. Like "burping" a baby, but a much harder pounding with alternating karate chops. So we did just that and it worked! When the crisis was over I told Gertrude that I knew she didn't want to go back to the hospital, but she had really scared me. She said "shit, you were scared? I was the one who was choking!"

"Holding Cancer in My Hand"
A Learning Everywhere® Experience

At about 3:00 a.m., after having gone back to bed, I awoke to the Home Health Aide who stood at the bottom of the stairs softly calling my name. You can imagine what I was thinking. When I answered she told me Gertrude wanted me. When I got to her bed side, I asked "are you alright?" She said "yes". She wanted me to know she had been talking to God. I asked her what they had been talking about and she told me she couldn't tell me, "its private." When I laughed and questioned "then why did you wake me up?" She said, "I just wanted you to know everything is going to be alright and it will be over soon."

While Gertrude was talking to God again later that morning, I talked to four Doctor's Offices and two transportation services trying to coordinate appointments. While doing this I got a call to confirm a Positron Emissions Tomography (PET) scan two days later. I told the Cancer Care Center we would be there and that Gertrude was being transported by ambulance on a stretcher. The Nurse then asked "can she get in a wheel chair? " I couldn't answer as my response surely would have been openly sarcastic! If she could get in a wheel chair, would she be transported via stretcher? She then asked if she could "get from a wheel chair into the trailer" where the PET scan would occur? I told her a chair lift would be required. She then asked "can she get from the chair to the table? I said, "with assistance." I then told her we knew about the pre-examination requirements, but 32 ounces of fluid prior to the scan was

Written by Sheila Stenhouse Lee

"Holding Cancer in My Hand"
A Learning Everywhere® Experience

not going to happen. She told me "she has to get to the bathroom to empty her bladder." I told her Gertrude was on a catheter and I didn't think that would be necessary. She gave the go ahead for the appointment, but I was concerned that we would never even get from the door to the stretcher, and I was right.

"Holding Cancer in My Hand"
A Learning Everywhere® Experience

Chapter IX

"Yard by yard life is hard................Inch by inch life's a cinch"

(Author Unknown)

    For many days after Gertrude came home we struggled to figure out how to administer medication. Four to six different medications up to four times daily (none of which were provided in liquid form, something the Medical Professionals forgot to mention) and to provide nourishment to a woman with esophageal cancer.

    It was on this day as we dressed Gertrude, I realized how thin she was. Her eye lids and lips were turning black from the lack of nutrition and it was all I could do to choke back the tears. Even so, through her own initiative, Gertrude sat with her feet over the side of the bed and then asked if she could sit in a chair. Shortly thereafter she wanted to get back in the bed, it was too much, but clearly she wasn't ready to give up. We were both inspired and pleased that she had tried and I realized a plan of action was required, but I wasn't sure what to do. Then feeling exhausted and overwhelmed Gertrude raised her hands and I heard her pray: "Father, I stretch my hands to thee." That was a prayer she said numerous times a day, she said it in good times and bad, everyone who knew her, had heard it. Once when her granddaughter was a mere toddler she came into the room

Written by Sheila Stenhouse Lee

"Holding Cancer in My Hand"
A Learning Everywhere® Experience

after being out of earshot for far too long. Gertrude asked her what she had been doing. Her brown eyes got all big and wide and she said "Father, I stretch my hands to thee." We laughed for a long time about that one! It was so funny because her granddaughter knew even at that age that whatever she had been up to she was going to need "back up." At that point I realized too now more than ever we were going to need some back up. There was only so much we could do.

Gertrude's inability to eat was one of the biggest issues we faced. I wanted her not to be sick anymore and I told her so. I realized for a person struggling to swallow we had to minimize the number of times a day when that needed to happen. So we concluded, myself and the Home Health Aides, that medications should be blended with food. The first attempt, with a menu of Gertrude's choosing, was not a success. She tasted the medicine right away. Gertrude then asked for something different without meds, but I asked the Home Health Aide to slip some in as the last dose literally didn't go down. After the first spoonful Gertrude accused us of being dishonest and we admitted that we had mixed the second dish with meds, too. She pushed the dish away and refused to eat another bite. I'm not really sure that the taste mattered so much as we were not doing as we were told. On several occasions during this time, Gertrude often reminded me that she was still and would always be my mother.

Written by Sheila Stenhouse Lee

"Holding Cancer in My Hand"
A Learning Everywhere® Experience

It was hard to watch a woman who has always been so formidable just wasting away. Her mind and wit were still sharp, but she was just so tired and weak and I realized at that point she weighed less than 100 lbs. During a quiet conversation that day, I told her I was keeping a journal to help process my thoughts about this experience and might possibly write a book someday. Because Gertrude was so private and proud I didn't know how she would respond. Initially she didn't say anything, but as there were daily frustrations, issues and her health continued to decline, one day she simply said out of nowhere "write the book!" So I do so with her blessing.

Written by Sheila Stenhouse Lee

Chapter X

"I'm so tired, but I must keep going"

Four days later, when the visiting nurse and Nurse Jane Fuzzy Wuzzy arrived at Gertrude's house they both commented how painfully thin she was. I was at a lost as how to proceed and they both recommended it was time for a feeding tube. I called the cancer doctor's office and asked how to arrange that. They told me to call the gastroenterologist who Gertrude saw in ICU and schedule the appointment. I got the sense if we had not initiated this it never would have happened. I got the number and explained this was "an emergency" as Mom was literally starving to death. As God would have it the gastroenterologist had just had a cancellation for the following morning at 9:00 a.m. I called and canceled the PET scan and changed the time of the ambulance to coincide with the new appointment. Gertrude agreed it was necessary because of her weakened state, but she also told me that after this procedure she didn't want any further anything that couldn't be provided at home.

The Home Health Aide and I traveled to the hospital with Gertrude for the outpatient procedure, the insertion of a Percutaneous Endoscopic Gastrostomy (PEG) tube. The gastroenterologist came to me shortly after the procedure and explained that everything had gone well, but the tube could not be used for 24 hours. At that time 1 ½ oz. of Ensure, an over the counter liquid

"Holding Cancer in My Hand"
A Learning Everywhere® Experience

nutrient, could be given every hour during a 12 hour period (for a total of 18 liquid oz.). If Gertrude wanted anything orally she could have it too. He recommended admitting her so the hospital staff could monitor Gertrude overnight to make sure the insertion was draining okay and that there was no sign of infection. In addition, Gertrude would have nutrients via an IV drip until she was discharged the next morning. I knew it would be a hard sell. It was supposed to be an outpatient procedure, but if staying overnight was for the best, we would do it. Even if it meant spending another night by her side sleeping in a hospital chair.

  The Wound Specialist consulted with us and advised that the sore on her back was superficial, but as Gertrude would need to be on her backside all night to receive the feeding tube nutrients the bedsore would become a pressure point where further breakdown would occur. She gave us two chair cushions as well as an order for an alternating air mattress to use at home.

  It was a horrible night. Around 11:00 p.m. Gertrude's pressure spiked to 204 over 98. Not a surprise as Gertrude had not had any medications all day. The doctor was called and authorization was given to administer her medication orally, but as it wasn't in liquid form Gertrude couldn't swallow it. An LPN came in once during the night to check her oxygen, temperature and pressure and once again it was high. She said she would check with the doctor again about more

"Holding Cancer in My Hand"
A Learning Everywhere® Experience

medication. At that point Gertrude asked to be repositioned and the Nurse said she had to get some help and she would be right back. After about 20 minutes I went in search of her to advise I could help. Right outside Gertrude's door was another nurse who was sitting outside a patient's room reading her mail. I realized she was on a 24 hour watch, but when I said hello she didn't even respond. When I got to the nurse's station there was absolutely no-one there and as I went back to Gertrude's room I realized almost every room that had a patient in it had a call button light that was lit. A few minutes later I saw a shadow in the hall and the LPN was talking to the night watch nurse and I told her I would help her. While we were repositioning Gertrude I asked what the other person was doing besides reading her mail. She informed me she couldn't leave her post. It was clear she was aggravated by my question (how dare I ask) and her handling of Gertrude which I'm sure was a direct result was a little clumsy, but I didn't say anything as I realized we are at the hospital's mercy. She never came back with any additional medications, but I don't know for sure if the doctor was contacted, what he said or if they just conveniently forgot about us.

The next morning, as Gertrude was waiting to be discharged a nurse came in with a nutrition supplement. Gevity. When I asked what it was she told me it was the supplement for the feeding (PEG) tube. She wanted to show us how to use it, even though at home we would have a pump. This was already totally different from

"Holding Cancer in My Hand"
A Learning Everywhere® Experience

what we had been told by the gastroenterologist the previous day, but luckily I thought to call the Senior Home Health Aide to come into the hospital to observe. While we waited for her to arrive I asked, quite confused as the gastroenterologist had told us to use Ensure, where we would get this nutrition supplement called Gevity and the pump. The nurse advised that the doctor needed to call in the prescription. I suggested that they go ahead and make those arrangements as Gertrude was being discharged that day. Then the Wound Specialist came in and reminded us Gertrude needed an air mattress too. I asked again that they go ahead and make those arrangements as Gertrude was being discharged that day. Finally the Discharge Planner came in and said that they were making arrangements for the Gevity, the pump, and the mattress, but because it would take most of the rest of the day they would like to keep Gertrude another night. Gertrude had been a real trooper up to that point, but I knew this was not going to fly. Gertrude sat up in bed and she said "No, I'm going home." I left Gertrude with the Senior Home Health Aide early that afternoon. I hated to do it, but I had to be at the house to receive the equipment that was now being sent "rush delivery" because no one on the medical staff thought to plan ahead. I ask, wouldn't it have been better to cancel if there have been complications during the night rather than wait almost 24 hours to get the process started? Or was it better to incur even more hospital expenses due to poor planning?

Written by Sheila Stenhouse Lee

"Holding Cancer in My Hand"
A Learning Everywhere® Experience

I waited at the house that afternoon with Gertrude's friend who had stopped by to visit her. Few people had any idea what was going on as things were constantly changing. While we sat and waited for the delivery of medical equipment I kept a look out through the sun room window of the new fence and a shed installation that Gertrude insisted be completed in the backyard. Even in her weakened state she wanted the house to look nice.

Although the medical supply company that was to deliver the mattress called at about 2:30 p.m. and said they were on their way, they didn't actually arrive until about 5:10 p.m. which was minutes before Gertrude arrived home via ambulance. Gertrude was so mad at me because I had left her alone (albeit with the Sr. Home Health Aide) at the hospital and it made me feel bad. During these times I often struggled with loyalties vs. logistics, as I could not be everywhere all the time, and most of the time Gertrude wanted me with her. She never said it, but I'm sure she was scared.

My final frustration that day was when the ambulance driver came into the house, looked into Gertrude's bedroom from the doorway and asked if there was any other way to get her into the room. (It was very narrow.) When I told him "no" he promptly told me they couldn't get her in there even though it was the same exact way they had brought her in and out several times before. I wanted to suggest they try a window, but I

Written by Sheila Stenhouse Lee

"Holding Cancer in My Hand"
A Learning Everywhere® Experience

feared my sarcasm would be lost on him and he would actually try. After saying my own prayer, I explained that she had been transported in and out of that same room three times prior via ambulance and I was sure they could do it again. After they got Gertrude settled and I signed the paperwork I told him to have a little faith next time.

That evening around 7:00 p.m., a visiting nurse arrived to show 3 of the 5 Home Health Aides who would be attending to Gertrude how to use the feeding tube and wean her up to the necessary portions. They did a great job and after a day or two Gertrude's coloring got better and her energy level began to increase.

I was overwhelmed and I, too, was losing weight. Most of my time was either spent with Gertrude who I didn't like to eat in front of or driving from the medical supply store, to the pharmacy, to the market, to the library (to print documents or send emails) or the office supply store (to send faxes). I was literally surviving on milkshakes from the corner dairy barn.

Addition to her five Home Health Aides, Gertrude had routine visits from nurses, a wound specialist, a dietician and a physical therapist. Needless to say her days were pretty full and her spirits were good. So it was out of the blue when I came to town a few days after to take her to the Cancer Care doctor that she proudly announced she was not going to see her doctors anymore.

Written by Sheila Stenhouse Lee

"Holding Cancer in My Hand"
A Learning Everywhere® Experience

I begged and cajoled, but there was no changing her mind. She was done and the appointment was canceled. I asked if that included her primary care doctor (Shorty) too and she told me to never mention his name in her presence again. Now mind you this is a doctor who when contacted about pain medication prescribed 5mg of Ambien. I've never been pre-med, but if you watch TV, listen to the radio or read at all, you know Ambien is a sleeping pill and 5mg wouldn't even put a toddler to sleep. So after a few nights of Gertrude having just enough Ambien to make her agitated and restless, I pulled it from her list of medications. So when she said she wouldn't see Shorty again, she got no argument out of me. But at that point I had to call the Cancer Care Doctor too. She said she understood and would put us in touch with Hospice.

So again I was shocked the next morning when Gertrude had the Home Health Aides to wake me to say she wanted to go to the hospital. I asked her if there was something wrong, she said "No." I asked her if she was in pain, she said "No." I told her if we went to the hospital they would poke and prod her and I wouldn't be able to just bring her home whenever she wanted. She said she knew that, but she just wanted to go to the hospital. I told her that when I called 911 I would have to tell them something. "What should I say?" She said "tell them you found me and I can't talk, I can't speak." I said, what?" She said "tell them you found me and I can't talk, I can't speak." As the realization of what she was

"Holding Cancer in My Hand"
A Learning Everywhere® Experience

saying hit us like a ton of bricks we both started laughing hysterically. Then as her laughter quickly turned to tears, she said "oh I don't know, I'm just sick of this bed and these walls. I want to get out of this room." The gravity of the situation had gotten to us, so I said "oh, okay" and with that I mobilized the Home Health Aides. By using a portable ramp that one of them was kind enough to lend us, we put her in a transport chair and rolled her to the sun room. She got to see the new fence and shed which made her cry and then we moved Gertrude to one of her favorite wing backed chairs and there we sat. Well I laid on the sofa, while she sat in the chair and we watched T.V. and talked. It was like old times. Gertrude soon got tired and asked to go back to bed, but it was one of the best times we had in a long time and ever would again.

Chapter XI

"Coke or Pepsi"

We did see the gastroenterologist again because I was insistent that we needed to make sure that everything was ok with the feeding tube. Gertrude agreed to go this one last time, but said "No more doctors!" A Home Health Aide and I transported Gertrude by car and all together we went to and fro in a little more than an hour. Fortunately the gastroenterologist said that everything was fine and through the tube feeding Gertrude was getting about 1,700 calories per day. She only needed to come back on an as-needed basis. Some days her progress made me forget she was dying.

Nonetheless, we had some real challenges when the feeding tube, which was the only means to provide nourishment, as well as medications, would clog or fail. Along with the Home Health Aides we learned to use the mortar and pestle to grind Gertrude's medication, add some warm water, than administer it through a big plastic syringe directly into the tube. The pump had to be adjusted periodically to ensure Gertrude wasn't getting too many calories as her body was slowly shutting down and not able to digest things as well. Sometimes the pump would fail and a technician from the medical supply company would have to be called in for maintenance. In addition, sometime there was just plain "operator error." For example, once when I was trying to change the bag, I squeezed too hard and myself, Gertrude, the walls and the drapes got drenched. Not one of my finest moments.

All of these things were learned on our own through trial and error without much coaching or guidance from her medical doctors. However, the best information we ever received (over the phone) from an Emergency Room nurse when the feeding tube had clogged for the 3rd or 4th time that day was priceless. The nurse suggested we put some Coke or Pepsi into the syringe and just keep pushing until the clog was dislodged. It was like waiting for a balloon to burst, but it worked! As a result, a bottle of soda remained a regular part of the medical supplies.

Over the next few months Gertrude's condition deteriorated and she often begged for the hot metal rod, the bed sore, in her back to be removed. Hospice came every day and tended to the wound, which eventually required packing, but it never healed. Gertrude would often get agitated and beg the Lord to take her, but in the same breathe tell us she didn't want any morphine because she didn't like being so out of control. Gertrude got confused and would often say "she didn't know where she was" which was hard to understand as it was the same house, same bedroom she had slept in for 55 years. We put cards that people had sent on the walls to give the room some definition, but kept everything else in place so as not to add to her confusion.

"Holding Cancer in My Hand"
A Learning Everywhere® Experience

I had to make some tough calls, the loyalty vs. logistics thing again. No morphine. Recognizing that there might be conflicting opinions on this, I hid it for use only during the direst of times. During those times the Home Health Aides had to call me first because no-one knew where I had put it. Every time I went to Gertrude's I would move it again. Knowing that being with Gertrude in her condition for extended periods could be taxing for the most professional of the Home Health Aides, I limited shifts to eight hours for her safety and their sanity. Gertrude had forewarned me there would come a time when she would be incommunicable. But when, in that state, I heard her blood curdling scream as Hospice attempted to change her catheter it was clear what she was trying to say. I asked them stop and remove it. After all we had 24 hour care and if she wet the bed they would simply have to clean it and her up. Finally, Hospice advised that feeding and water should cease to be most humane to Gertrude and we complied. But after several days, Gertrude was still with us and I asked the Home Health Aides to give her whatever her body could hold. I don't know if it made any difference, but I felt it was the right thing to do.

I remember clearly the day I realized I had held cancer in my hand. Gertrude often drooled because she could no longer swallow. The thick purplish phlegm that poured from her lips was so very cold. As I would sit with her and wipe her mouth I realized the phlegm was as

Written by Sheila Stenhouse Lee

"Holding Cancer in My Hand"
A Learning Everywhere® Experience

cold as any ice I had ever held. That's when I realized……… I was holding cancer in my hand.

These final months where troubling in that as Gertrude struggled to be free and yet hang on, I questioned what else she wanted, needed us to do. I remembered that when she was able, just a few months prior, we had talked about the fact that clearly God was not ready for her yet and either she still had something left to do or He was giving us time to get prepared. One friend even mentioned "God is probably working on her personalized Tootsie Roll® factory and/or her shoe closet," but I still wasn't sure. I often sat by her bed side and held her hand, sang Christmas Carols, or prayed. I remember the last time we were together, I whispered in her ear with tears in my eyes that I just didn't know what else to do and that we would all be alright. Her eyes became fixated in a stare and she laid that way for several hours. She eventually closed her eyes and never opened them again.

Written by Sheila Stenhouse Lee

"Holding Cancer in My Hand"
A Learning Everywhere® Experience

Written by Sheila Stenhouse Lee

Epilogue

Gertrude died on December 10, 2010. Almost 6 months to the day of her diagnosis. She was not the type to wait around, but more likely she, like my Dad, was probably trying to ensure we had time to gather and to get back home ....as she knew well there would be no limit to the grieving period.

"Holding Cancer in My Hand"
A Learning Everywhere® Experience

Written by Sheila Stenhouse Lee

"Holding Cancer in My Hand"
A Learning Everywhere® Experience

Self Help

This portion of the book is intended to help those who aren't sure where or when to start when a loved one is faced with a health crisis. On the following pages you will find sample outlines, contracts, checklists and other documents to help you navigate all that has to be done, things you may want to do, or things that will happen to you.

Many of the documents going forward are only legally binding if sanctioned by a legal representative in the state in which they are drafted.

"Self Help" is not intend to constitute legal advice or legal information. The author makes no claims, promises or guarantees about the accuracy, completeness, or adequacy of the information contained herein. The resemblance of sample documents, checklist, contracts or comments related to formal legal agreements is purely coincidental.

Chapter XII

Vial of Life

Every home needs a "vial of life." It's a repository for all the information that needs to be accessible should a patient need to be moved in an emergency. It is a packet of information that contains all of the patient's important documents and necessary items. It should contain a copy of the Health Care Proxy, a DNR, patient identification, insurance cards, a list of medications, house and or car keys.

The "vial of life" should be kept on a top shelf or butter dish of the refrigerator door in a clear plastic bag for easy visibility. Why the refrigerator? Because every home has one. Where is it? In the kitchen. It can be easily found.

When there is an emergency and there is a lot of commotion, it is invaluable to be able to go to one central location to get everything you, the hospital, and the patient will need.

Chapter XIII

Pre-Paid Funeral Plans

To help relieve their families of some of the burial decisions and expense, an increasing number of people are planning their own funerals, designating their funeral preferences, and sometimes even paying for them in advance.

Gertrude had pre-paid for her funeral at the time of my father's death more than 25 years prior. That included embalming, interment, head stone engraving, funeral services, flowers, limousines and the casket. At the time of her passing the only decisions that remained were type of flowers and casket color.

Often Gertrude would say to me "I have a pre-paid funeral plan and I want you to spend every dime." What I didn't know was the plan she purchased accrued interest over those 25 years since its original purchase and there was an additional amount of money above and beyond what had initially been invested.

These plans are pretty common and available upon request. Some plans require payment in full at the time of purchase, others require payment over time. However, in most instances interest will only begin to accrue once the plan is paid in full.

Chapter XIV

(Sample) Last Will and Testament

I, _____ (Name) of _____ (City, State), declare this to be my Last Will and Testament, hereby revoking all other Wills and Codicils heretofore made by me.

ARTICLE I: IDENTIFICATION OF FAMILY (LIST)

ARTICLE II: FUNERAL PROVISIONS

ARTICLE III: PAYMENT OF TAXES

ARTICLE IV: TANGIBLE PERSONAL PROPERTY

ARTICLE V: SPECIAL BEQUESTS

ARTICLE VII: POWERS OF PERSONAL REPRESENTATIVE

ARTLE VIII: OPERATION OF BUSINESS

ARTICLE IX: DESIGNATION OF PERSONAL REPRESENTATIVE

ARTICLE X: WILL CONTEST

ARTICLE XI: MISCELLANEOUS PROVISIONS

ARTICLE XII: TERMS AND DEFINITIONS

ARTICLE XIII: CHOICE OF LAW

ARTICLE XIV: SAVINGS CLAUSE

ATTACHMENTS:

- (A) Real property transactions
- (B) Tangible or intangible personal property transactions
- (C) Stock and bond transactions
- (D) Commodity and option transactions
- (E) Banking and other financial institution transactions
- (F) Business operating transactions
- (G) Insurance and annuity transactions
- (H) Estate, trust and other beneficiary transactions
- (I) Claims and litigation
- (J) Personal and family maintenance
- (K) Benefits from Social Security, Medicare, Medicaid or other governmental programs, civil or military services
- (L) Retirement transactions
- (M) Tax matters
- (N) Gifts and other estate planning

IN WITNESS WHEREOF, I have hereunto signed my name this ____ day of _____, ____.

_____

(Name)

"Holding Cancer in My Hand"
A Learning Everywhere® Experience

_____STATE OF (Name)
/_____CITY OF (Name)

Notary Public

My Commission Expires:

Written by Sheila Stenhouse Lee

"Holding Cancer in My Hand"
A Learning Everywhere® Experience

Chapter XV

(Sample) Health Care Proxy

_____ (Name) hereby appoint:

Agent(s): _____
Name of Agent

_____
_____
Address of Agent

_____
Telephone Number of Agent

as my health care agent to make any and all health care decisions for me except to the extent I state otherwise.

This health care proxy shall take effect in the event I become unable to make my own health care decisions.

Note: Although not necessary, and neither, encouraged or discouraged, you may wish to state instructions or witnesses, and limit your agent's authority. Unless your agent knows your wishes about artificial nutrition and hydration, your agent will not have the authority to

"Holding Cancer in My Hand"
A Learning Everywhere® Experience

decide about artificial nutrition and hydration. If you choose to state instructions, wishes or limits, please do so below:

If a situation should arise in which there is no reasonable expectation for my recovery from extreme physical or mental disability, I direct that I will be allowed to die and not to be kept alive by medications, artificial means, life support equipment or "heroic measures." I do, however, ask that medication be mercifully administered to me to alleviate suffering.

This statement is made after careful consideration and is in accordance with my convictions and beliefs. I urge those concerned to take whatever action necessary, including legal action, to fulfill my wishes and directions.

I direct my agent to make heath care decisions in accordance with my wishes and instructions as stated above or as otherwise known to him or her. I also direct my agent to abide by any limitations on his or her authority as stated above or as otherwise known to him or her.

In the event the person I appoint in unable, unwilling or unavailable to act as my health care agent, I hereby appoint:

"Holding Cancer in My Hand"
A Learning Everywhere® Experience

Agent(s): _____
    Name of Agent

    _____
    _____
    Address of Agent

    _____
    Telephone Number of Agent

Written by Sheila Stenhouse Lee

"Holding Cancer in My Hand"
A Learning Everywhere® Experience

Chapter XVI

(SAMPLE) Do Not Resuscitate Order (DNR)
_____ (state of authority)

Person's Name

_____

Date of Birth   -

_____

Do not resuscitate the person named above.

Physician's Signature

_____

Print Name

_____

License Number

_____

Date

_____

It is the responsibility of the physician to determine, at least every 90 days, whether to continue this order as appropriate, and to indicate this by a note in the person's medical chart. The issuance of a new form is NOT required, and under the law this order should be considered valid unless it is known that it has been revoked. This order remains valid and must be followed, even if it has not been reviewed within the 90 day period.

"Holding Cancer in My Hand"
A Learning Everywhere® Experience

Chapter XVII

(SAMPLE) Contractual Agreement For Independent Home Care Services

_____ (Health Care Manager) on behalf of _____ (Patient) is providing this contract to _____ (Name of Provider) Independent Home Care Services.

1. Scope of Work
This Agreement outlines the responsibilities for both parties.

2. Performance Agreements
  2.1. _____ (Health Care Manager) **agrees:**
   - To serve as a Point of Contact (POC) should _____ (Name of Provider) Independent Home Care Services or _____ (Patient) require.
   - To coordinate payment of invoices submitted by _____ (Name of Provider) Independent Home Care Services.

  2.2. _____ (Name of Provider) Independent Home Care Services **agrees**:
- To provide twenty four (24) hour Home Health Aide Services to _____ (Patient) seven (7) days per week. Duties include assistance with Bathing,

Written by Sheila Stenhouse Lee

"Holding Cancer in My Hand"
A Learning Everywhere® Experience

Toileting, Dressing, Meals, Medicine, Daily Exercise, and Light Housekeeping to include: bathroom, kitchen (un/loading the dishwasher), laundry and garbage/recycling.

- To advise _____ (Patient) or _____ (Health Care Manager or POC) should circumstances in the home or related to the current medical condition change.
- To maintain all certifications, licenses and insurances necessary for fulfill the terms of this agreement.
- To ensure all staff arrive on time and never leaves the home until the next staff member arrives as scheduled and to conduct all activities in a professional and courteous manner.
- To not substitute, sub-contract or reassign services to any other party for any reason without express permission from _____ (Patient) or _____ (Health Care Manager).
- To refrain from disclosing information of a personal nature regarding the home, location or medical condition of _____ (Patient) to anyone for any reason without express permission from _____ (Patient) or _____ (Health Care Manager).

3. Terms and Conditions

3.1. Period of Performance

The base period of performance for this agreement will commence on day, mm/dd/yyyy and terminate at a mutually agreed upon future date.

3.2. Place of Performance

The work shall be performed at the primary

residence of _____ (Patient) at - _____ (Street Address, City, State, and Zip Code).

3.3. Performance Criteria

_____ (Health Care Manager) in conjunction with _____ (Patient) will monitor the performance of _____ (Name of Provider) Independent Home Care Services staff, to ensure ongoing quality and consistency in services provided.

3.4. Termination Clause

Either party may terminate this agreement, in writing with no requirement of stated cause two (2) weeks from notification of termination. This contract will be automatically terminated should either party cancel three (3) consecutive days unless there are extenuating circumstances and both parties agree.

3.5. Rate Schedule

_____(Name of Provider) Independent Home Care Services will be compensated at a rate of $XX.00 (XX Dollars) per hour Monday at 7:00 a.m. through Friday at 7:00 p.m.

_____(Name of Provider) Independent Home Care Services will be compensated at a rate of $XX.00 (XX Dollars) per hour Friday at 7:00 p.m. through Monday at 7:00 a.m.

_____(Name of Provider) Independent Home Care Services may not invoice for canceled sessions and there is no reimbursement provided for time or expenses related to travel.

3.6. Invoicing

_____ (Name of Provider) Independent Home Care Services will submit one invoice for the total number of twenty four (24) periods provided within a thirty (30) day period. Invoices must be received no later than thirty (30) days following the period of performance. Invoices may be submitted by email, fax, or postal mail to:

Mail: _____ (Health Care Manager)

Street Address
City, State, Zip Code

E-mail: xxxxxxxxxxxx@xxxxxxxx.com

Fax: xxx-xxx-xxxx

Invoices must include Name, Social Security Number or Employer Identification Number, Dates of Service, Location of Services, Hours, Rate, and Payment Address.

Payment will be remitted within fifteen (15) days of receipt of invoice.

4. Authorization

Signature below indicates acceptance of the terms described in this Agreement.

_____
(Name of Provider)

_____
Date

_____
Independent Home Care Services (Health Care Manager)

_____
Date

Independent Home Services

_____
Street Address

_____
City, State, Zip

_____
SSN or EIN

Chapter XVIII

(SAMPLE) Contract for in Home Physical Therapy

_____ (Health Care Administrator) on behalf of _____ (Patient) is providing this contract to _____ (Service Provider) on behalf of _____ (Company name and full address).

1. **Scope of Work**

    This Agreement outlines the responsibilities for both parties.

2. **Performance Agreements**

    2.1. _____(Health Care Administrator) agrees:

    - To serve as a Point of Contact (POC) should _____ (Service Provider) or _____ (Patient) require.

    - To coordinate payment of invoices submitted by _____ (Service Provider).

    2.2. _____(Service Provider) agrees:

    - To provide a schedule for _____(X) hour physical therapy session (s) to _____(Patient) _____(X) per week at a time to be arranged by - _____ (Service Provider) at a mutually agreeable time.

- To advise _____ (Patient) or _____ (Health Care Administrator) should circumstances in the home or related to the current medical condition change.

- To maintain all certifications, licenses and insurances necessary for fulfill the terms of this agreement.

- To arrive on time as scheduled and to conduct all activities in a professional and courteous manner.

- To refrain from using a substitute, sub-contractor or to reassign services to another party for any reason without express permission from _____ (Patient) or _____ (Health Care Administrator)

- To refrain from disclosing information of a personal nature regarding the home, location or medical condition of _____ (Patient) to anyone for any reason without express permission from _____ (Patient) or _____ (Health Care Administrator), except as deemed medically necessary and in accordance with the Health Insurance Portability and Accountability Act (HIPPA) of 1996.

3. Terms and Conditions

3.1. Period of Performance

The base period of performance for this agreement will commence on _____ day (mm/dd/yy) and terminate at a mutually agreed upon future date. If at any time during the course of care _____ (Patient) is admitted to any inpatient facility or home care agency, this agreement can be placed in suspension until she is discharged from that care. At such time this agreement can be reinstituted as written unless any changes in performance are deemed necessary and agreed upon by all parties.

3.2. Place of Performance

The work shall be performed at the primary residence of _____ (Patient) at _____ (Address, City, State, and Zip Code).

3.3. Performance Criteria

_____ (Health Care Administrator) in conjunction with _____ (Patient) will monitor the performance of _____ (Service Provider) to ensure ongoing quality of service and consistency in services provided.

3.4. Termination Clause

Either party may terminate this agreement, in writing with no requirement of stated cause, one week from receipt of written notification of termination.

This contract will automatically be terminated should either party cancel three (3) consecutive sessions unless extenuating circumstances require and both parties agree.

3.5. Rate Schedule

_____ (Service Provider) will be compensated at a rate of $XX.XX (XX Dollars) per hour.

_____ (Service Provider) may not invoice for cancelled sessions and there is no reimbursement provided for time or expenses related to travel.

3.6. Invoicing

_____ (Service Provider) will submit one invoice for the total number of Physical Therapy sessions provided within thirty (30) day period. Invoices must be received no later than thirty (30) days following the period of performance.

Invoices may be submitted by e-mail, fax, or postal mail to:

Mail: _____ (Health Care Administrator)

_____ (Address)

"Holding Cancer in My Hand"
A Learning Everywhere® Experience

_____ (City, State, Zip Code)

email:_____@XXX.com

Fax: _____ (NUMBER)

Invoices must include Name, Social Security Number or Employer Identification Number, Dates of Service, Location of Services, Hours, Rate, and Payment Address.

Written by Sheila Stenhouse Lee

"Holding Cancer in My Hand"
A Learning Everywhere® Experience

Chapter XIX

Important Contacts

(Include name, address, phone number, and email)

Personal
Family Friend
Neighbor
Clergy

Household Services
Heating, Ventilation and Air Conditioning
Electrical
Snow Removal
Lawn Care
Plumber

Prescriptions
Pharmacy / Drug Company
Medical Supplies
Lab Corporations

Physician Information
Primary Doctor
Specialists
Dentist

Estate
Lawyer
Mortuary

"Holding Cancer in My Hand"
A Learning Everywhere® Experience

Chapter XX

List of Medications

As prescriptions are filled, which sometimes is initiated by pharmacies automatically, please check for accuracy and question substitutions. Mistakes happen.

Date	Prescribed Medication	Strength	Prescribing Physician	Dosage	Caution(s)

Written by Sheila Stenhouse Lee

"Holding Cancer in My Hand"
A Learning Everywhere® Experience

Chapter XXI
Prescription Schedule

Many stores have multi-dosage prescription trays. The tray should be filled by the same person every week. This person should keep abreast of all prescriptions, changes and generic brands used so that medications can be properly administered.

Prescription Schedule	Sun	Mon	Tues	Wed	Thurs	Fri	Sat
5:00 a.m.							
6:00 a.m.							
7:00 a.m.							
8:00 a.m.							
9:00 a.m.							
10:00 a.m.							
11:00 a.m.							
12:00 p.m.							
1:00 p.m.							

Written by Sheila Stenhouse Lee

"Holding Cancer in My Hand"
A Learning Everywhere® Experience

Time							
2:00 p.m.							
3:00 p.m.							
4:00 p.m.							
5:00 p.m.							
6:00 p.m.							
7:00 p.m.							
8:00 p.m.							
9:00 p.m.							
10:00 p.m.							
11:00 p.m.							
12:00 p.m.							
1:00 a.m.							
2:00 a.m.							
3:00 a.m.							

Written by Sheila Stenhouse Lee

"Holding Cancer in My Hand"
A Learning Everywhere® Experience

Chapter XXII

Items to Have on Hand

Antiseptic
Adult diapers
Cane
Catheter bags and tubing
Circulations socks
Disposal sheets
Favorite candy
Favorite music
Feeding tubes
Feeding tube pump
Gauze
Gloves
IV pole
Lotion
Medical bed
Medications
Medical syringes
Oxygen tubes, tanks and masks
Portable commode
Saliva suction device
Swabs
Talc
Walker
Wheel chair

Chapter XXIII

Health Care Journal

As a way to maintain a health care record it is helpful to compile notes on the patient's care, medical condition and daily routines. A simple journal noting date and time of entry is helpful to determine what has transpired since the last review. At a minimum these entries should be made every 12 hours. The following items are things you may want to include.

1. Medications
2. Meals
3. Outputs
4. Doctor Appointments
5. Visitors
6. Daily Activity
7. Medical Emergencies

"Holding Cancer in My Hand"
A Learning Everywhere® Experience

Chapter XXIV

Accounts Payable

Routine/Regular (as applicable)
    a. Alarm Company
    b. Ambulance Service
    c. Cable
    d. City Recycling
    e. Gas and Electric
    f. Home Health Aides
    g. Hospital
    h. Insurance(s)
    i. Lawn Care (Seasonal)
    j. Medical Alert System
    k. Mortgage/Rent
    l. Physicians
    m. Prescriptions
    n. Property Taxes
    o. School Taxes
    p. Snow Removal (Seasonal)
    q. Telephone
    r. Trash Removal
    s. Water Bill

Based on Need
    a. Electrical
    b. Heating, Ventilation and Air Conditioning
    c. Medical Supply Company

Written by Sheila Stenhouse Lee

       d. Plumbing
       e. Tax Preparation

One Time Payments
       a. Church
       b. Clergy
       c. Estate Sales
       d. Funeral Home
       e. Probate Attorney
       f. Realty Company
       g. Settlement Attorney
       h. Title Attorney

"Holding Cancer in My Hand"
A Learning Everywhere® Experience

Chapter XXV

Important Papers

In preparation for the liquidation of the estate a "resource book" is helpful and should include a copy of the Will or agreements of disbursement of personal property (consignment, antique dealers), pictures of residence and contents, probate information, death certificate, preplanning funeral arrangements, pension services, and real estate contracts, etc.

1. Auto Title
2. Birth Certificate
3. Death Certificate
4. Financial Records
    a. Savings
    b. Checking
    c. IRAs
    d. Bonds
    e. CDs
    f. Safety deposit box
5. Fine Art Receipts
6. Insurance Policies
7. Jewelry Receipts
8. Marriage Certificate
9. Military Discharge papers
10. Property Deed
11. Service Repair Receipts
12. Tax Records

Written by Sheila Stenhouse Lee

"Holding Cancer in My Hand"
A Learning Everywhere® Experience

Written by Sheila Stenhouse Lee

"Holding Cancer in My Hand"
A Learning Everywhere® Experience

Glossary

The glossary is intended to be an quick reference for all of the terms that may get batted back and forth between family, bankers and lawyers while trying to sort out who is responsible for what, and who has authority to make what decisions.

"The Glossary" is in no way intended to represent a complete list of terms and conditions that may be needed. The author collected simple and general terminology from a variety of resources for the sole purpose of reference material for the reader. It should be duly noted that further consultation with financial and legal experts is likely required.

Glossary

A Trust- A surviving spouse's portion of an A-B Trust, i.e. Marital Trust or Survivor's Trust.

A-B Trust – A Trust with a provision for your surviving spouse, while keeping control over who will receive your assets after your spouse dies, and permitting a couple to leave up to the combined amount of your estate tax exemptions to your Beneficiaries or estate-tax free.

Administration – A court supervised distribution of an estate during probate.

Administrator – A person named by the court to represent a probate estate when there is no Will or the Will did not name an Executor. (Female is Executrix.) A male or female may also be called Personal Representative.

Alternate Beneficiary – Person or organization named to receive your assets if primary Beneficiaries named in your Will or Trust die before you do, are unable or refuse to take the property.

Ancillary Administration – Additional probate proceeding conducted in another state. Typically required when you own real estate in another state that is not titled in the name of your Trust.

"Holding Cancer in My Hand"
A Learning Everywhere® Experience

Annual Exclusion – An amount you can give someone each year without having to file a gift tax return or pay a gift tax.

Assets – Includes anything you own, i.e. real estate, bank accounts, life insurance, investments, furniture, jewelry, art, clothing and collectibles.

Assignment – A transfers of your interest in assets to another.

B Trust – The deceased spouse's portion of an A-B Trust, i.e. Credit Shelter or Bypass Trust.

Basis – Purchase price of an asset. The value is used to determine gain or loss for income tax purposes.

Beneficiaries – The persons and/or organizations named in a Living Trust, who receive or benefit from the Trust assets after the death of the Trust Grantor.

Bequeath – To give personal property by will.

Bypass Trust – The "B" part of an A-B Living Trust related to assets in the Trust bypass federal estate taxes.

C Trust – See "QTIP."

Certificate of Trust – A Trust that verifies the Trust's existence, explains the powers given to the Trustee, and identifies the Successor Trustee(s). It does not reveal any information about the Trust assets, beneficiaries or other inheritances.

Children's Trust – If, when you die, a Beneficiary is not of legal age, the child's inheritance will go into this Trust. The inheritance will be managed by the Trustee you have named until the child reaches the age at which you want him/her to manage the inheritance. It is typically a Trust included in your Living Trust.

Codicil – A written change or amendment to a Will.

Co-Grantors – Two (2) or more persons who establish one Living Trust together.

Common Trust – One Living Trust established by two (2) or more individuals (usually a married couple).

Community Property – Assets a husband and wife acquire by joint effort during marriage if they live in a community property state. Each spouse owns half of the assets in the event of divorce or death.

Conservator – One who is legally responsible for the care and well-being of another person. If appointed by a court, the Conservator is under the court's supervision. May also be called a Guardian.

Conservatorship – A court-controlled program for persons who are unable to manage their own affairs due to mental or physical incapacity. (May also be called a Guardianship.)

Contest – To dispute or challenge the terms of a Will or Trust.

Corporate Trustee – A formal institution, like a bank or trust company that is serving as a Trustee.

Co-Trustees – Two (2) or more individuals who have been named to act together in managing a Trust's assets. A Corporate Trustee can also be a Co-Trustee.

Credit Shelter Trust – A "B" Trust in an A-B Living Trust because this Trust "shelters" or preserves the federal estate tax "credit" of the deceased spouse.

Creditor – A person or institution to whom money is owed.

Custodian – Person named to manage assets left to a minor under the Uniform Transfers to Minors Act. The minor typically receives the assets at legal age.

Deceased – One who has died. Also called decedent.

Deed – A document that transfers title of your real estate to another person(s). Also see warranty deed and quitclaim deed.

Disclaim – To refuse to accept a gift or inheritance so it can go to the recipient who is next in line.

Disclaimer – A denial or disavowal of any interest in or claim to the subject of the action, such as, renunciation of any title, claim, interest, estate or trust.

Discretion – Full or partial power to make a decision or judgment.

"Holding Cancer in My Hand"
A Learning Everywhere® Experience

Disinherit – To prevent someone from inheriting from you.

Distribution – Payments in cash or assets(s) to one who is entitled to receive it.

Durable Power of Attorney for Asset Management – A legal document giving another person full or limited legal authority to act on your behalf in managing your assets and affairs. This is valid through incapacity, but ends at death.

Durable Power of Attorney for Health Care – A legal document that gives someone else the authority to make health care decisions for you in the event you are unable to make them for yourself. Also called a Health Care Proxy or Medical Power of Attorney.

Equity – The current market value of an asset less any loan or liability.

Estate – Assets and debts left after an individual's death.

Estate Taxes – Federal or state taxes on the value of assets left at death. Also called inheritance taxes or death taxes.

Executor – Person or institution named in a Will to carry out its instructions. Also called a Personal Representative.

Family-Owned Business Estate Tax Exemption – An additional estate tax exemption for family-owned businesses and farms that qualify.

"Holding Cancer in My Hand"
A Learning Everywhere® Experience

Federal Estate Tax Exemption – Amount of an individual's estate exemption from estate taxes.

Fiduciary – Person having the legal duty to act primarily for another's benefit. Implies great confidence and trust, and a high degree of good faith.

Funding – The transfer of assets to your Living Trust.

Gain – The difference between what you receive for an asset upon sale sold and the purchase price. This is used to determine the amount of capital gains tax due.

Generation Skipping Transfer Tax – A tax imposed on any generation-skipping transfer at a flat rate computed with reference to the maximum federal estate rate applicable at time of transfer.

Gift – A transfer from one individual to another without fair compensation.

Gift Tax – A federal tax on gifts that exceed a certain dollar amount made while you are living.

Grantor – The person who transfers or grants property rights by means of a trust instrument or some other document.

Gross Estate – All of a person's property before debts, taxes and other expenses or liabilities are deducted.

GST Trust – Any trust having beneficiaries who belong to two (2) or more generations younger than the grantor.

"Holding Cancer in My Hand"
A Learning Everywhere® Experience

Guardianship – See "Conservatorship" or "Durable Power of Attorney for Health Care."

Heir – One who is entitled by law to receive portions or all of your estate contents.

Holographic Will – A handwritten Will. It may include a Homestead Exemption which may include a portion of your residence (dwelling and surrounding land) that cannot be sold to satisfy a creditor's claim while you are living.

Incompetent – Unable to manage one's own affairs, either temporarily or permanently, i.e., lack of legal capacity.

Independent Administration – A form of probate intended to simplify the probate process by requiring fewer court appearances and less court supervision.

Inheritance – The assets received from someone who has died.

Intangible Property – Property which cannot be touched nor realized with the senses, such as a legally enforceable right by the holder of a promissory note or a bond.

Inter vivos – Is created while you are living.

Intestate – Deceased without a Will.

Irrevocable Trust – A Trust that cannot be changed (amended) or canceled (revoked) once it is set up.

"Holding Cancer in My Hand"
A Learning Everywhere® Experience

Issue – All persons who descended from a common ancestor, i.e. a broader term than children.

Joint Ownership – When two (2) or more persons own the same asset.

Joint Tenants with Right of Survivorship – A form of ownership in which the deceased owner's share automatically and immediately transfers to the surviving joint tenants.

Liquid Assets – Cash and other assets that are converted into cash.

Living Probate – The court-supervised process of managing an incapacitated persons assets.

Living Trust – A written legal document that creates an entity to which you transfer ownership of your assets. Contains your instructions for managing your assets during your lifetime and for their distribution upon your incapacity or death. Avoids probate at death and court control of assets at incapacity.

Living Will – A written document in which a person states in advance his or her wishes regarding the use or removal of life-sustaining or death-delaying procedures in the event of a terminal illness or injury.

Marital Deduction – A deduction on the Federal Estate Tax Return that lets the first spouse to die leave an unlimited amount of assets to the surviving spouse free of estate taxes. In the event no other tax preparation, and the surviving spouse's estate is more than the amount of the

Written by Sheila Stenhouse Lee

federal estate tax exemption at the time of his/her death, estate taxes will be due.

Marital Trust – See "A Trust."

Medicaid – A federally funded health care program for the poor, minor and disabled children.

Medicare – A federally funded health care program for persons over age 65 who are covered by Social Security or Railroad Retirement benefits.

Minor – One who is under the legal age for an adult (usually age 18 or 21).

Net Estate – The value of an estate after all debts, taxes and expenses have been paid.

Net Value – The current market value of an asset minus any loan or debt.

Payable-on-Death Account – See "Totten Trust."

Per Capita – A way of distributing your estate so that surviving descendants will share equally, regardless of their generational relationship.

Per Stirpes – A way of distributing your estate so that your surviving descendants will receive only what their immediate ancestor would have received if he/she had been living at the time of your death.

Personal Property – Movable property.

"Holding Cancer in My Hand"
A Learning Everywhere® Experience

Personal Representative – Another title for an Executor or Administrator.

Pour Over Will – A short Will that states that any assets left out of your Living Trust will become part of (pour over) your Living Trust upon death.

Power of Attorney – A legal document giving someone legal authority to act on your behalf. This typically ends at incompetency (unless it is a durable power of attorney) or death.

Probate – The legal process of validating a Will, paying all debts, and distributing assets as designated after death.

Probate Estate – Assets that go through probate after you die. This usually includes assets in your name and those paid to your estate. Does not include assets owned jointly, payable-on-death accounts, insurance and other assets with beneficiary designations.

Probate Fees – Court costs and legal, executor and appraisal fees charged when an estate goes through probate. Usually paid from assets in the estate before the assets are fully distributed to the heirs.

Qualified Domestic Trust (QDOT) – Allows a non-citizen spouse to qualify for the marital deduction.

Qualified Terminable Interest Property (QTIP) – A Trust that delays estate taxes until the surviving spouse dies.

Qualifying Subchapter S Trust (QSST) – A Trust that meets IRS qualifications.

Quitclaim Deed – A document that allows you to transfer all your interest in real property via title without making guarantees.

Real Property – Land and property that is permanently attached.

Recorded Deed – A deed that has been filed with the county land records creating a public record of all changes in ownership of property in the state.

Revocable Trust – A Trust in which the person setting it up retains the power to change (amend) or cancel (revoke) the Trust during his/her lifetime.

Separate Property – All assets you acquire prior to marriage and assets acquired by gift or inheritance during marriage.

Separate Trust – A Trust established by one person regardless of their marital status.

Settle an Estate – The process of handling the valuation of assets, payment of debts and taxes, distribution of assets to Beneficiaries after someone dies.

Settlor – See "Grantor."

Special Gifts – A separate listing of special assets that will go to specific individuals or organizations after your incapacity or death.

Special Needs Trust – Allows you to provide for a disabled loved one without jeopardizing government benefits.

Spendthrift Clause – Protects assets in a Trust from a beneficiary's creditors.

Stepped-up Basis – New basis for assets when transferred by inheritance (through a Will or Trust) as of the date of the owner's death. If an asset has appreciated above what the owner paid for it, the new basis is called a stepped-up basis. A stepped-up basis can save a considerable amount in capital gains tax when an asset is later sold by the new owner.

Successor Trustee – Individual or institution named in the Trust document who will take over should the first Trustee die, resign or otherwise become unable to act.

Surviving Spouse – The spouse who is living after one spouse has died.

Survivor's Trust – See "A Trust."

Tangible Property – Property which can be touched or realized with the senses.

Taxable Gift – The value of the gift is applied to your federal gift and estate tax exemption, and no gift tax is required to be paid until the exemption has been exhausted.

Tenants-by-the-Entirety – A form of joint ownership applicable in some states between husband and wife. When one spouse dies, his/her share of the asset transfers to the surviving spouse.

Tenants-in-Common – A form of joint ownership in which two (2) or more persons own the same property. At death his/her share transfers to his/her heirs or devisees.

Testamentary Trust – A Trust created in a Will effective at death of the will maker.

Testate – A person who dies with a valid Will.

Title – A legal document that proves ownership of an asset.

Totten Trust – A bank account that will transfer to the named Beneficiary when the account was established. This timing can be modified based on the inclusion of "transfer on death (TOD)," "in Trust for (ITF)," "as Trustee for (ATF)" and "pay on death (POD)."

Transfer Tax – Tax on assets when they are transferred from one to another.

"Holding Cancer in My Hand"
A Learning Everywhere® Experience

Trust – A fiduciary relationship in which a trustee holds legal title to assets for the benefit of certain persons or entities.

Trust Company – An institution that specializes in managing Trusts.

Trustee – Person or institution who manages and distributes trust assets according to the instructions in the formal Trust documentation.

Trustor – See "Grantor."

Unfunded – A Living Trust is unfunded if assets have not been transferred.

Unified Credit – A specified dollar amount allocated to each taxpayer used to offset gift and estate taxes that would otherwise be owed.

Uniform Transfer to Minors Act (UTMA) – State specific law enacted that allows for designations of assets to a minor by appointing a Custodian.

Warranty Deed – Document that allows you to transfer title to real estate. The title being transferred is clear (free of any encumbrances).

Will – A written document with instructions for disposing of assets after death. Enforceable only through the probate court.

"Holding Cancer in My Hand"
A Learning Everywhere® Experience

Written by Sheila Stenhouse Lee

"Holding Cancer in My Hand"
A Learning Everywhere® Experience

ABOUT THE AUTHOR

With Gertrude's encouragement Sheila expanded Sheila Lee & Associates, LLC – Learning Everywhere® from a consultancy to a full fledge business in 2005 (www.learningeverywhere.com).

Although her time and attention to Learning Everywhere® was greatly diminished during Gertrude's illness, Sheila would have had it no other way, has no regrets (well just one) and would do it all over again given the chance. Sheila resides in Baltimore, MD with Gertrude's words of wisdom, memories and mementos all around her.

She is a member of New Psalmist Baptist Church where upon hearing Bishop Walter Scott Thomas say "Father I Stretch My Hands to Thee" she knew she was home.

On daily basis Sheila is heard repeating the prayer in her home, in her office, in her car, or on a plane. Everywhere, all the time, in good times and bad. Thanks Mom!

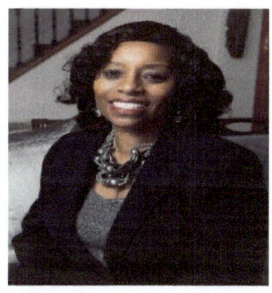

Written by Sheila Stenhouse Lee

www.ingramcontent.com/pod-product-compliance
Lightning Source LLC
Chambersburg PA
CBHW040808200526
45159CB00022B/57